Intermittent Fasting

An Easy Guide to Living a Longer, Healthier Life While Burning Fat and Losing Weight

© Copyright 2018 - All rights reserved.

The contents of this book may not be reproduced, duplicated or transmitted without direct written permission from the author.

Under no circumstances will any legal responsibility or blame be held against the publisher for any reparation, damages, or monetary loss due to the information herein, either directly or indirectly.

Legal Notice:

This book is copyright protected. This is only for personal use. You cannot amend, distribute, sell, use, quote or paraphrase any part or the content of this book without the consent of the author.

Disclaimer Notice:

Please note the information contained in this document is for educational and entertainment purposes only. Every attempt has been made to provide accurate, up to date and reliable, complete information. No warranties of any kind are expressed or implied. Readers acknowledge that the author is not engaging in the rendering of legal, financial, medical or professional advice. The content of this book has been derived from various sources. Please consult a licensed professional before attempting any techniques outlined in this book.

By reading this document, the reader agrees that under no circumstances is the author responsible for any losses, direct or indirect, which are incurred as a result of the use of information contained within this document, including, but not limited to, —errors, omissions, or inaccuracies.

Table of Contents

INTRODUCTION

I would like to take this opportunity to thank you for purchasing this book: "Intermittent Fasting: An Easy Guide to Living a Longer, Healthier Life While Burning Fat and Losing Weight."

Have you wondered why there is so much hype about intermittent fasting? A lot of well-known celebrities across the world like Hugh Jackman, Chris Martin and The Rock have vouched for this method of fasting. Today, intermittent fasting is gaining popularity and people are turning to this fasting method for weight loss. There have been close to 246,000 searches for Intermittent Fasting on the world's best online search engine – Google. The search volume clearly shows the growing popularity of this fasting method. Nutrition experts and scientists look at it as the next big thing, which will help people lose weight and keep their BMI (Body Mass Index) in check. More articles and books have been published on this trending topic – Intermittent Fasting.

It is strange to believe that one of the most efficient and best ways to transform your health is to deprive yourself of your basic need – food. However, there is evidence to prove that fasting can definitely help improve the health of both your mind and body. There are several different types of fasting, which can range from extensive fasting for longer periods to consistent diet control (watching out for calories!) to interval fasting to periodic or intermittent fasting.

Of all these fasting methods, intermittent fasting is considered to be one of the most popular and effective methods to lose weight and improve health. Different groups of bio-hackers obsessed with self-optimization meet once a week to collectively break their fast in Silicon Valley. And also there are few executives in companies like Facebook who claim that fasting has helped them lose weight and become more energetic.

In this book, we will discuss the history of fasting and the benefits of intermittent fasting on brain health and longevity. The chapters in this book will help you understand the rules of the different fasting methods and the various types of intermittent fasts that you can participate in. The chapters will also talk about how to get started with intermittent fasting and frequently asked questions (FAQs) on this topic.

I hope this book serves as an informative and interesting read to you!

Happy Reading!

CHAPTER ONE:

Fasting Throughout History

Fasting is an ancient tradition and has been in practice since the beginning of time. It is a time-tested approach to cure medical conditions and for the wellness of your body. Fasting helps not only with weight loss but also with:

- Longevity
- Reversing the aging process
- Improved concentration
- Insulin resistance
- Alzheimer's
- Diabetes

The main question on weight loss is not – what should you eat? It is – when should you eat?

Almost all food we consume increases the insulin levels in our body to a certain degree, but there are some foods that are better than others. If you eat the right food, your insulin levels will not shoot up. The key to preventing insulin resistance is to maintain low levels of insulin.

Fasting

Fasting is not new, so it definitely cannot be called a new diet trend. Our ancestors have tried it for hundreds of years. It is advisable to concentrate on the primitive healing traditions of the past rather than trying out a new alien diet pattern. Fasting is the solution that was adopted by every religion and culture on Earth. Therefore, it is considered the most ancient tradition followed by humans.

Everyone has his own definition of fasting, which ultimately results in a lot of misunderstanding. The word fasting originated from the Anglo Saxon language – it was originally referred as faest, which means fixed or firm. During the early days, people refrained from eating food during specific periods. When a person deliberately avoided food, it was referred to as fasting.

In general, fasting refers to refraining from consuming any type of food completely. But when you look at it from a religious stance (most religions for that matter), fasting refers to avoiding specific foods. For instance, a person can eat fruit during the fasting period in certain religions.

So, when a person only consumes juices during the fasting period, he is said to be on a juice fast, but basically, it needs to be referred to as a juice diet.

When you look at it on a broader perspective, fasting is considered as negative nutrition convincing the organism to survive on stored sustenance.

When you mention to your parents or friends that you plan to fast, you get an eye-roll from them as a response. This is followed by a couple of questions. Why do you want to starve yourself? Why do you want to inflict damage on your otherwise healthy body?

Fasting Vs. Starving

No! Fasting is not starving. Both are entirely different concepts. Starvation is the complete absence of food, and you don't do it deliberately. It is not controlled. People who starve will have no idea when they will get their next meal. On the contrary, fasting is intentionally controlling food or refraining from having food for health, religious or various other reasons.

Do you know the difference between suicide and natural death? It is impossible to confuse the two terms. Similarly, fasting and starving are entirely different. Fasting might be done for a period of time – few hours, a day, a week or even months together. To be precise, fasting is an object of your regular life. For instance, breakfast actually means breaking the fast, i.e., a meal that breaks the fast – which you do every day.

The word starve comes from the old English word steorfan – it means mortality or pestilence. When you mention that you are going to starve yourself, it literally means that you are going to die. It is because when you starve, you don't know when you will get your next meal. Sometimes you might not get meals for days on end. In such cases, all the nutritional reserves in your body are used to keep you alive and then one fine day it will get completely exhausted, which leads to death.

In the case of fasting, you enable your body to use its nutritional reserves only during the fasting period. Because once your fasting cycle is over, you get back to the feast mode. So, your nutritional reserve gets stocked up again. But, in the case of starvation, the entire nutritional reserve is exhausted, and the tissues start to break down.

History of Fasting

As mentioned earlier, fasting has a long history – it is the oldest and one of the most ancient healing practices. Hippocrates, widely known as the Father of modern medicine, prescribed and supported the practice of fasting among all his other treatments. He also advocated the consumption of apple cider vinegar. He wrote – *'To eat when you are sick is to feed your illness.'* He lived between 460 and 370 BC.

Plutarch, a Greek historian and writer, also had the same opinion as Hippocrates. He mentioned that it is better to fast for a day instead of using medicine. He lived between AD 46 and AD 120. The famous Greek philosopher Plato and his student Aristotle were also ardent supporters of fasting.

According to the ancient Greeks, medical treatment should be found in Mother Nature. Animals don't usually eat when they are sick. Similarly, humans don't feel like eating when they aren't feeling well. This is the reason fasting is referred to as using the physician within. The reason humans, cats and dogs become anorexic when they are sick is due to their fasting instinct, which exists in the genes. Are you confused? Think of the last time you felt ill. Did you feel the urge to eat when you were sick? It must have been the last thing you wanted to do. Therefore, fasting is the universal human instinct to many different health conditions.

Fasting is said to improve cognitive abilities, and it is no surprise that the ancient Greeks had a similar belief. When was the last time you had a huge feast? A delicious lip-smacking meal that almost burst your stomach? What were the after-effects of the meal? Did you feel energetic or enthusiastic? I don't think so! You may have wanted to sleep for a while due to a drowsy feeling. Why does this happen? The blood is pushed to your digestive system, as it needs more support in the digestion process due to the huge influx of food. This will ultimately result in less flow of blood to the brain, which results in food coma (sleep state due to consumption of a large amount of food).

There were so many other intellectual personalities who were equally good advocates of fasting. The founder of toxicology – Philip Paracelsus quoted – *"Fasting is the greatest remedy – the physician within."* He was one of the three fathers of modern Western Medicine (the other two were Galen and Hippocrates). Our very own Benjamin Franklin, one of the founding fathers of the United States, mentioned fasting as one of the best medicines. He said – *"The best of all medicines is resting and fasting."* He lived between 1706 and 1790, and donned many different hats – author, politician, scientist, civic activist, inventor, etc.

Fasting was practiced as a part of religious rituals in almost all major religions in the world. Fasting is referred to as purification or cleansing in a spiritual context. The practice of fasting gradually developed among different cultures and religions. They had their own methods and rules attached to it. It was not considered harmful but something that will fundamentally benefit the human spirit (mind) and body.

Religions and their fasting methods

In Buddhism, the followers have food in the morning and fast from noon until the next morning. This is their regular routine. They also have strict water-only fasts for a couple of days or sometimes even for weeks.

The Greek Orthodox Christians followed a variety of fasting methods for over 180 to 200 days in a year.

Muslims fast during the Ramadan month – they consider that period to be holy. They fast from sunrise to sunset, i.e., they have food before the sun rises and then fast until the sunsets. They break their fast after sunset. According to their beliefs, Prophet Muhammad inspired them to fast on Mondays and Thursdays every week.

Researchers and experts have studied the Ramadan fasting periods as they differ from the usual fasting protocol. During the fasting period, they are not allowed to have any form of fluids – no water either. This sometimes results in mild dehydration too. Recent studies showed that the daily intake of calories during this period significantly rises, as they are allowed to eat before sunrise and after sunset. Since most people usually eat large amounts of food before sunrise and after sunset, they don't really get the benefits of fasting.

Based on these facts, it is obvious and clear that fasting is an age-old custom. When you already have the three most influential people to have ever lived (Jesus Christ, Buddha, and Prophet Muhammad), agree to the concept of fasting and its benefits, do you still think it is a harmful ritual?

History of Intermittent Fasting

Fasting is the most simple and definite method that can be followed when compared to most other traditional dieting techniques. In all probability, you have already practiced it – maybe unintentionally – by skipping dinner or breakfast. Whenever you skip a meal, you get into the fasting mode.

In olden times (the hunter-gatherer days), when the ancient cavemen were looking for food, they were in the fasting state. Agriculture began as a way of life during the later stages of civilization. Then, gradually, the concept of civilization – kingdom, tribe or specific society, came into existence. During these different eras, fasting never faded, as whenever there were food scarcities or natural calamities, people fasted to ensure their supplies lasted longer. Castles and cities stored grains for winter. When the rains failed, it was famine – people fasted to ensure their stored food could last until it rained again.

When the concept of civilization was practiced, religions taught people to share and care. They brought in certain traditions and beliefs. Along with all these, fasting also became a part of religious customs (in almost all the religions). Each had their own concepts and rules. Hinduism used fasting as a mechanism to respect their deities or for personal penance.

Fasting was observed during auspicious days or festivals. People in Judaism observed fasting during their holy day – Yom Kippur. They refrained from eating, drinking, working, wearing leather and having intercourse during this 25-hour period.

Today, fasting would mean the following:

- Skipping breakfast
- Having no food after dinner
- Skipping dinner and then breaking fast with your first meal the next day (usually breakfast)

Our modern era of processed food has entirely changed the way food is consumed. Our unhealthy food habits have already led to a series of health issues that our society is facing today. Though intermittent fasting is an age-old practice, it has gained popularity among people because of its various health benefits. Your body naturally cleanses, repairs the tissues and regenerates cells for best performance when you fast.

CHAPTER TWO:

Losing Weight and Burning Fat

Most weight loss diets are complex with many rules. It is fortunate that one of the most popular fasting methods to lose weight doesn't have too many rules or conditions. Intermittent fasting keeps it simple – it is a dieting pattern where you tactically skip one or more meals for a particular period.

Intermittent fasting is not about cutting calories from your meal, but instead skipping an entire meal. This is why it is considered as one of the easiest dieting patterns. The reasons behind the growing popularity of intermittent fasting are:

- Simple eating pattern
- Effectiveness to lose belly fat and reduce weight
- Other health benefits

Intermittent fasting and weight loss

Intermittent fasting, as the name suggests, is a dieting pattern where you have to fast for a specific period in a day. The fasting usually lasts between 16 to 20 hours, and you eat during the other 4 to 8 hours of the day. The fasting period is referred as the fasting window and the time you eat is known as the eating window. During the fasting window (the period you fast), you are allowed to have fluids (water, black coffee, herbal tea, etc.).

You can see better results when you spend more time fasting on a daily basis. There is no specific chart – you can fast as frequently as you prefer. The more you fast, the more effective the result.

When you follow Intermittent fasting, you gain more health benefits apart from weight loss. How does your body lose weight when you fast? Your body uses the stored body fat (nutritional reserve) for energy. This results in burning all the unwanted calories. When you burn calories in this way, you lose weight and also burn the excess fat. This will help you get a lean physique, and you will also feel healthy and energetic, as the body uses the excess body fat (stored fat) for energy. This is because it doesn't get energy from the food intake since your food intake is restricted.

Intermittent fasting helps your body to optimize the release of the major fat burning hormones – especially insulin and HGH (Human Growth Hormone) – the two most important ones. Human Growth Hormone is responsible for switching on your body's fat burning system. Your body starts to burn all the excess fat to give you the energy to carry on with your regular work (routine).

Studies show that fasting increases the production of the human growth hormone (HGH), by 2000 percent in men and 1300 percent in women.

Intermittent fasting also has a major influence on the other important hormone – insulin. It helps to keep the insulin levels steady and low, which is key to losing excess weight or avoiding extra fat from becoming accumulated in the body. Foods rich in processed carbohydrates and simple sugar accumulate more body fat. It is therefore advisable to avoid these foods as it causes the insulin levels to skyrocket and then crash whenever you eat them. This will result in excess fat accumulation in your body instead of burning it as energy.

When your insulin levels go up, you end up with health issues like obesity, Type II diabetes, and various other chronic health conditions. Intermittent fasting is the solution to all these problems. Clinical studies have proven that 15 days of consistent intermittent fasting helps to balance the insulin levels. Your body stays in a fat burning state giving you more energy all through the day.

Strategies of Intermittent Fasting

Intermittent fasting naturally reduces calorie intake

For a weight loss diet to work, there should be an overall reduction in the total calorie intake. The process of burning more calories than you actually consume is referred as a caloric deficit. A caloric deficit will lead to weight loss. Intermittent fasting does this naturally.

When you skip an entire meal, you don't take in any calories for that period. This, of course, means that you don't have to worry about the calories when you eat. For instance, when you skip your regular breakfast of lemon juice and toast sandwiches, you might save about 400-500 calories each day. Now, let's say, you are planning to reduce 1500 calories per day, you already saved 33 percent of the calories right away by skipping a meal.

Even if you eat two large meals (600 calories each) after skipping breakfast, you only consume 1200 calories, which is not too high.

Intermittent fasting helps to lose the extra fat

When you say you want to lose weight, you essentially mean that you want to lose your body fat. The fact is — nobody wants to lose their muscle mass or water content in the body. But most weight loss diets do this — it first cuts the carbs and then pulls out the water from the body. Ultimately, this weight loss regimen doesn't serve any actual purpose.

Research has shown that fasting helps the body to lose more fat content and less water content or muscle mass. On the contrary, most of the other weight loss diet patterns do the opposite. The study was able to prove that intermittent fasting helped people reduce 4 to 7 percent of their waist size in a period of 24 weeks, i.e., they lost belly fat – the most difficult fat to burn in the body.

More studies proved that alternate day fasting (a type of intermittent fasting) reduced around 3.8 kg body fats on an average.

Intermittent fasting helps maintain muscle mass

The main problem with most weight loss patterns is that you tend to lose both fat and muscle. To experience healthy weight loss, it is important to maintain the muscle mass of your body. This is because muscle maintenance is elementary to make sure the metabolic rate of your body doesn't go down too low.

If you don't maintain muscle and concentrate only on fat loss, then you might get back the lost fat once you stop the diet pattern. A review shows that overweight people can lose body fat and maintain muscle through fasting as compared to the usual calorie-restriction diets. There was another study which showed that around 25 percent of the lost weight was muscle mass in the usual calorie-restriction diets. While on intermittent fasting, (which involved calorie restrictions), only 10 percent muscle mass was lost.

Nevertheless, a good protein diet and strength training are the two most important aspects to building muscle mass.

Intermittent fasting works well when your weight gain is at the highest

You don't gain weight overnight – it is a gradual process that happens over the years. Though there is no consistency in the amount of weight we gain, it usually skyrockets during holiday breaks like Christmas and Thanksgiving. Research shows that around 50 percent of weight gain happens between November and January in a year. So, if you keep checking on your weight during the festive seasons every year, you don't need to worry about weight gain. Unfortunately, it is not easy to do, as you might look like a fool when you count your calories and macronutrients during your Christmas feast. But, there is a better way! You can observe intermittent fasting during such occasions. For instance, you can skip your breakfast and have a sumptuous Christmas lunch followed by a light dinner.

The basic thing here is to miss one or two meals on the day you are planning to feast. This way, you don't really need to worry about missing out on your favorite food.

Intermittent fasting doesn't give you hunger pangs or yo-yo effects

What is yo-yo effect? The yo-yo effect, also called weight cycling, is the recurring gain and loss of weight over time. When you introduce your body to a restrictive diet, it causes a shift in your hunger hormones. Due to this, you might end up with uncontrollable food cravings and severe hunger pangs.

Intermittent fasting will not cause the yo-yo effect as the fasting and eating pattern is broken into intervals. This means such a fasting method can cut calories from your body without making you feel hungry.

Intermittent fasting can be a game changer for you if you:

- Want to lose belly fat
- Can skip meals without making a fuss
- Want to spend less time cooking and cleaning (On a lighter note!)

How effective is intermittent fasting to lose fat?

Intermittent fasting encourages your body to burn more fat. Your blood sugar rises after you finish your meal. The blood sugar and the glycogen (stored carbs) in your body is the energy (your body burns), which is responsible to keep you alive and functioning in good health. So, when you don't eat anything for a longer period, your body's blood sugar and the stored carbs go down. When this happens, your body has no choice but to begin burning the stored body fat for energy.

Your body fat is nothing but the accumulation of all the excess calories that get stored in the body every time you overeat.

The body takes all these excess calories and stores them as body fat (nutritional reserve) to use as a backup energy source when:

- You become calorie-deficit due to heavy exercising or when you eat less.
- Your body is forced to burn all these excess calories, which are stored as body fat as there are not enough carbs or blood sugar to burn when you are fasting for more than 14 hours.

So, when your body fat gets burned for energy, you naturally start to lose weight as all the excess calories are getting burned.

When you combine intermittent fasting with a proper exercise plan, you tend to lose more fat and body weight thereby giving you a lean physique.

You lose fat faster when you,

- Fast for 14 to 20 hours per day
- Eat less during your weight loss diet pattern
- Combine exercising and fasting

Your metabolic rate increases when you observe intermittent fasting. This is because when your energy levels go down, along with your blood sugar levels, your body counter-reacts by releasing more adrenaline (norepinephrine). This gives you more energy and keeps you focused on your regular work routine. Since your body releases adrenaline, it forces your body to burn all the accumulated fat to provide you with energy. These stored fats are mostly found in the hips, belly and thighs.

It is true that intermittent fasting usually targets the belly fat area. It is extremely difficult to lose belly fat because the abdominal region has more alpha-2 receptors (they slow down fat burning) than the beta-2 receptors (they speed up fat burning). When you observe intermittent fasting, your insulin level goes down, which closes down the A2 receptors (as they can't work well without insulin). This will activate the B2 receptors in your abdominal region allowing your body to burn the excess fat in the belly. The increased blood flow to the belly area makes it easier for the fat-burning hormones to do their job well.

It is possible to reduce the last bit of fat your body has accumulated, through intermittent fasting. And this fasting method is more essential for women as they have more fat (or A2 receptors) in their thighs, butt and hips. As mentioned earlier, the growth hormone naturally increases due to intermittent fasting and helps burn more fat. This also stops you from eating more calories as you skip one or more meals that reduce the calorie intake.

CHAPTER THREE:

Your Brain and Intermittent Fasting

There is new research that indicates fasting can considerably reduce the effects of aging on the human brain. Intermittent fasting observed on a regular basis can have a strong anti-inflammatory effect on the complete body. Most of the leading scientists accept the fact that this form of fasting can help improve the brain's health condition. It is one of the main approaches that can be followed to maximize the functionality of the brain.

Studies conducted by researchers at the National Institute of Aging in Baltimore proved the positive effects fasting could have on the overall health condition of the brain. It is made clear by the head of the Institute's Laboratory of Neurosciences, Professor Mark Mattson, that these benefits (on brain health) are more to do with the intermittent fasting periods and not just the restriction of calories.

Role of intermittent fasting for super brain power

Fasting has exceptional and unique benefits for the various functions of the brain. Intermittent fasting is said to boost the brainpower and improve the cognitive function. It induces neuronal autophagy, which permits the brain cells to recycle and repair by themselves for the brain's optimal functionality. This cleansing process of the brain cells is referred as autophagy activation. This is not just restricted to humans but to all mammals on this Earth. When the body is severely deprived of calories, most of the major organs will start to shrink (in size) – except for the testicles and the brain.

Autophagy activation

Autophagy is the natural way for the body to cleanse itself from the inside out. When you train your body to do this, you are doing the best thing for your body. I am not trying to sound scary but, to be precise – your body will eat itself. That is, the active cells in your body kill the other diseased cells, regenerate them and repair the entire system. Autophagy plays a fundamental role in your body's ability to repair, regenerate and detoxify itself.

When you activate autophagy in your body, you optimize the functions of the brain, slow down the aging process and reduce inflammation. Multiple studies and research has already proved that it is possible to encourage autophagy inside the brain when you fast. This helps improve the brain structure, increase cognitive functions and neuroplasticity. Neuroplasticity permits the brain to change and adapt to situations continuously. It helps to make your brain more flexible to stress, which naturally adapts to the change. The best possible way to activate autophagy is through intermittent fasting (and, it has been clinically proven!)

Studies have shown that interfering with the neuronal autophagy can result in neurodegeneration of the brain. This means it can cause the brain to function inadequately and can stop you from performing your best.

Brain-Derived Neurotrophic Factor (BDNF)

Intermittent fasting helps to increase a particular protein in the brain known as the brain-derived neurotrophic factor (BDNF). BDNF manages the formation of new neurons and is responsible for the development of synapses and different communication lines within the brain. When the BDNF level is high, it means your brain has healthy neurons and can help in better communication between the neurological cells.

When the BDNF level goes down, you might get affected by either of the following issues:

- Alzheimer's
- Loss of memory
- Dementia
- Other brain-related issues (which is mostly connected to the processing of the brain).

Studies show that observing intermittent fasting for 16 to 18 hours can boost the growth hormone (HGH) levels by 50 to 100 percent. Another study has shown a boost of BDNF levels by 400 percent if one observes fasting for 36 hours. Asthma patients are highly benefitted by intermittent fasting due to the anti-inflammatory effect. Preliminary reports on people who have Parkinson's and Alzheimer's have shown good results. BDNF interacts with the parts of your brain that are responsible for controlling memory, cognitive function and learning. This protein (BDNF) not only protects your brain cells but also is responsible to stimulate the growth of new brain cells. BDNF is also referred as the Miracle-Gro for the brain.

Ketones and BDNF

Intermittent fasting is said to improve a person's mood and memory. Often, people mention that they feel more energetic and focused when they fast. When your body enters the fasting state, the ketogenic phase gets triggered. This, in turn, causes the release of BDNF which is naturally linked to memory and learning.

Ketogenesis is the process where your body turns to the stored fats for energy thereby processing the fat into ketones. These ketones can feed your brain by easily crossing the bloodstream to reach the brain. This will result in more productivity, energy, and mental sharpness.

It is possible to improve your brainpower by creating more brain cells. Dr. Mark Mattson, a Neurology professor at John Hopkins University, has indicated that fasting can increase the rate of neurogenesis in the brain. Neurogenesis is the process through which new nerve tissues are developed, and brain cells are grown.

The brain performance, focus, memory and mood increase when neurogenesis is high. Researchers used the 16:8 schedule (a type of intermittent fasting) for a study and were surprised to see the increased stimulation in the production of new brain cells.

You will by now be clear that intermittent fasting impacts the functions of the brain to a larger extent. Though not many are aware, the topic has been greatly researched, and the benefits of intermittent fasting have been identified for quite a long time now.

Think about how cave dwellers would have survived especially during the winter times when there was a scarcity of food. It would have been completely impossible for them to survive and look for food in the case of their normal brain functioning slowing down (especially during the times when food was limited). Therefore, it is evident that cognitive functioning of the brain is at its highest during the fasting period.

It was a common practice for the great philosophers and thinkers of ancient Greece to observe fasting in order to boost their mental alertness. This is the best historical example to prove that fasting has not just started recently but was in existence way before. The ancient Greeks followed fasting as a natural healing method to improve their cognitive ability and to sharpen one's mind.

Studies on the effect of intermittent fasting for better brain functionality

Professor Mark Mattson had given a speech for a TedX program on the subject of fasting and the effects it had on the brain. He mentioned about the studies where the participants were asked to observe fasting for specific intervals of time. The findings confirmed that it brought positive neurological changes to the brain. This had, in fact, improved the cognitive abilities and resistance to the stressful stimuli.

The studies also showed that restriction in the calorie-intake had helped with an anti-inflammatory effect within the brain. This also resulted in growth and production of new neurons that are responsible for memory and learning abilities.

Professor Mark Mattson went on to explain how the process of fasting challenges the brain. The brain responds to this challenge by adjusting to the response pathways that in turn help it to cope with the stress. He said that the reaction of the brain to intermittent fasting is similar to how it responds to regular exercises. Both these activities (exercise and intermittent fasting) increase the BDNF level (protein production) which, in turn, promotes the growth of neurons and increases communication between the nerve cells. Since it is responsible for the growth of neuron, it equally stimulates the ketone production and amplifies the number of mitochondria in the neurons. All these activities result in improved memory and more grasping power.

He also indicated that this method of fasting boosts the ability of nerve cells to repair the DNA. In case this happens, then it can be the starting point to cure medical conditions such as Dementia and Dystonia. According to Professor Mattson, there has been some research done in this arena, which has already given a positive outcome.

Almost all the findings show that intermittent fasting is not restricted only to weight loss but has improved effects on:

- Restricting heart disease
- Controlling diabetes
- Improving the brain functions
- Increasing the focus on learning
- Boosting the memory power

CHAPTER FOUR:

Cellular Repair and Longevity

Our bodies have developed a protective mechanism to adjust to the irregular phases of food scarcity and profusion. What led to this? Thousands of years of food shortage (the era of cavemen)! When the body is deprived of food, the cell membranes get more sensitive to insulin. This is particularly essential when food is limited, as it makes sure that every morsel of food is effectively utilized or stored.

But when there is excess food, the body makes the cell membranes less sensitive to insulin. This is necessary, as the stress of taking more calories needs to be avoided. When this happens, insulin levels go up, fat storage is more, oxidative stress is high, and the body's inflammatory condition also increases. Insulin boosts cellular division and reduces the risk of cancerous cell formation.

Today, the scenario is completely different – the food supply and its sources are abundant. We get to eat anytime we want. You have health experts recommending you to eat 5 to 6 small meals all through the day. But will this work well for the body? When you eat more meals in a day, your body receives the signal of excess food. This will hinder the key tissue repair hormones. These repair hormones have powerful anti-aging effects and when there is a hindrance in the process, then the body ages faster.

Fasting has been used for therapeutic and medical purposes for centuries.

Can fasting put an end to inflammation?

Inflammation is good when our body is trying to heal itself, but when it lasts for a longer period, inflammation can go bad. Inflammation for a longer period can lead to negative health conditions.

Many chronic health conditions such as arthritis, cancer, asthma, obesity and Crohn's disease (gastrointestinal) have constant inflammation involved. To add to this, inflammation is the main cause of most musculoskeletal disorders, such as lower back pain, short-term joint issues, osteoporosis and arthritis.

Recent studies show chronic inflammation can be cured by regular fasting. Leukotriene B4 (LTB4) has an important role in cellular processes that involves the release of enzymes, oxidative metabolism, stimulation of neutrophil aggregation and migration along with inflammation.

When you alter your lipid intake, it changes the phospholipid fatty acid composition of the cell membranes. This, in turn, impacts the predecessor substance content for producing the inflammatory leukotrienes. The food we eat plays a major role in chronic inflammation in the body.

For a study, 14 individuals affected by rheumatoid arthritis observed fasting for a week. They had inflammatory marker measurements taken before and after the fast. Fasting helped reduce the release of LTB4 from the rheumatoid arthritis neutrophils. It reduced the production of cytotoxins from the serum, which in turn changed the phospholipid fatty acid structure. The findings showed that the production of LtB4 was reduced, which confirmed that fasting, in fact, had the anti-inflammatory effects on the body.

Apart from slight weakness and dizziness, the fasting showed no other unfavorable effects. Many studies were successful in showing the importance of fasting to reduce calories without malnutrition. Chronic inflammation needs to be looked at seriously as it can impact every other part of the body which includes the brain. Chronic neuroinflammation can lead to Alzheimer's, depression and many neurodegenerative diseases.

How do you decrease inflammation in your body? A combination of proper diet, exercise and intermittent fasting (any form) can serve as the best tools to improve your health condition by reducing the inflammatory properties in the body. If you are looking to live a healthy and energetic life, then it is crucial to make the right change to your lifestyle.

Fasting for extended lifespan

Researchers and medical experts get excited when the research on fasting involves lifespan – or indeed extended lifespan!

Almost all of us have been in the habit of having three meals in a day, and this is, in fact, quite a recent development for us. This was not the case with our cavemen ancestors as their diet was completely unstable. They often had to go without food for longer periods, i.e., the fasting state. Fortunately, our bodies still adapt to the fasting routine.

Time and again, it has been proven that regular fasting can help improve the brain health, regulate blood sugar and protect the cell membranes in the body.

Genetic repair mechanism for longevity

Intermittent fasting serves as a switch to turn on specific genetic repair mechanisms that can boost cellular rejuvenation. This alteration of cell membranes allows certain cells to have a longer lifespan during times of food shortage. Repairing a cell needs less energy when compared to dividing and creating new cells. Therefore, it helps to shut down cancer cell formation and its production.

The genetic repair mechanisms get into active mode when the growth hormones (HGH) are released. HGH helps to generate physiological changes in metabolism that in turn helps to burn more fat. The amino acids and the proteins are used to repair the tissue collagen to improve muscle strengthening, better functioning of bones, ligaments and tendons. The secretion of growth hormones is also responsible to reduce wrinkles, heal cuts/burns quicker and improve the skin function.

HGH focuses on repairing tissues, working on the anti-inflammatory immune activity and efficient energy usage. On the contrary, Insulin concentrates on cellular division, pro-inflammatory immune activity and energy storage. If you take a closer look, the functionalities of HGH and Insulin are quite the opposite. Insulin dominates mostly as when the body condition demands the release of insulin (during intake of food rich in carbohydrates), the HGH hormone is repressed.

Intermittent fasting helps to increase tissue healing, boost immunity and reduce inflammation. Many people feel sick and dizzy when they have infections, and this built-in mechanism is the body's way to influence us to fast. When your body gets into the fasting state, it helps to produce the perfect environment to increase the natural immunity.

The best way to start fasting is by giving your body a 12-hour gap between dinner and breakfast daily. This 12-hour gap will allow the body 4 hours to digest and 8 hours for the liver to perform its function (finish the detoxification phase). Once you are able to follow this approach successfully, you can introduce fasting into your regular lifestyle. You can maybe fast for one day every week – the fasting window can be 16 to 18 hours.

Gradually, you can try the 24-hour fast once in a week regularly.

Intermittent fasting helps with the following:

- Reduces oxidative stress
- Improves insulin sensitivity
- Increases glucose uptake
- Decreases fat mass
- Reduces blood pressure

And all these factors help improve the health condition and increase longevity. As mentioned earlier, fasting can trigger autophagy, which helps the body to get rid of dead or weak cells, regenerate and recycle all the damaged proteins. This natural process (autophagy) is significant to prevent a series of diseases such as diabetes, liver conditions, cancer, autoimmune disorders, cardiomyopathy and many more.

Intermittent fasting for cancer

Preliminary human trials show that intermittent fasting can help reduce the risk of cancer or display a decrease in growth rate of cancerous cells. These studies show the following effects due to fasting:

- More production of tumor-killing cells
- Reduced production of blood glucose
- Triggering the stem cells to renew the immune system
- Balanced intake of nutrition.

Another research showed that chemotherapy with fasting could slow down the development of skin cancer and breast cancer. This was proved in the 2016 study. Fasting caused the body to generate high levels of CLPs (common lymphoid progenitor cells) and tumor-infiltrating lymphocytes. Lymphocytes are WBCs that can migrate into a tumor and kill them. CLPs are the precursor cells to these lymphocytes. It was in the same study the researchers came up with the following findings:

- Fasting between intervals can make cancerous cells sensitive to chemotherapy
- This protects the normal cells and promotes stem-cell production.

If you want to reduce the risk of cancer to your body, intermittent fasting will be the best chance you can take. This fasting method can reduce the body's insulin resistance and improve its sensitivity to insulin. This insulin resistance has already been linked to various types of cancers. Since fasting triggers autophagy (general and neuronal), it helps to clean up the unwanted cellular trash.

Though more human trials are required to prove the role of intermittent fasting in cancer prevention, the evidence in existence already shows some exciting favorable results.

Can fasting reverse type-2 diabetes?

The effectiveness of intermittent fasting has deep-rooted reasons that are complex and complicated. But there are few reasons that are merely common sense:

- Low blood sugar

When you eat, your blood sugar level rises. Simple science! So, naturally, when you are not eating, your blood sugar becomes lower. Now, here comes the magic! When you observe intermittent fasting, you tend to fast for 12 to 16 hours on an average. This permits your body to utilize the stored glucose in your system.

- Increase in insulin receptiveness

The insulin in your body works well when you fast as your cells are not overloaded with sugar. Insulin can easily do its job and move the sugar out of your blood.

- Low insulin levels

Now that your cells are receptive to insulin, the pancreas generates less insulin

- Reboots your pancreas

The pancreas produces insulin. When you have type-2 diabetes, your pancreas will have to do overtime to produce enough insulin to deal with the excess sugar in the blood. Studies have proved that intermittent fasting helps to reboot the pancreas and regenerate beta cells (to burn fat faster) effectively.

- Weight loss

Often, losing weight can be the first step to reversing type 2 diabetes. People have lost 3 to 8 percent of their body weight in three to 24 weeks through intermittent fasting.

- Increases body metabolism

When more calories (stored excess fat) are burnt, your body metabolism naturally increases.

Multiple studies have shown that intermittent fasting lowers blood sugar levels and that helps improve one's overall health condition. The World Journal of Diabetes published a study that mentioned its subjects (type-2 diabetes patients) observing short-term intermittent fasting on a regular basis. The findings confirmed the following:

- Reduction in body weight
- Improved glucose levels after meals

This method of fasting reduces stress, lowers blood pressure, reduces inflammation, improves lipid levels and shows improvement in glucose circulation. All these factors help reduce the risk of neurological disorders, cardiovascular conditions and cancer.

Therapeutic benefits

Physical benefits

Intermittent fasting is said to be effective to reduce seizures and brain damage caused by seizures. It also helps to heal rheumatoid arthritis apart from reversing diabetes. More research is starting to surface, which show the positive effects of alternate-day fasting (a type of intermittent fasting). This method helps to reduce the toxic effects caused by chemotherapy and also decreases the rate of disease/illness associated with cancer.

Spiritual benefits

Almost all the major religions in the world use fasting as a spiritual cleansing practice. It is quite interesting that all religions have their own set of beliefs and traditions, but when it comes to fasting, all of them unanimously follow fasting protocols to promote health, wellness and to heal. In some religions, fasting is looked at as a practice of penance. The result expected is wellbeing, self-love, peace and forgiveness. Such is the power of fasting!

Psychological benefits

Fasting helps to improve the willpower – this is because you are controlling your mind and training it to accept your decision to not eat. This is similar to your gym sessions where you train your muscles.

This training will help you to have control over your eating habits and that eventually helps to develop the power to control the various other aspects of your life. A recent study showed that women who observed intermittent fasting felt more positivity in their lives in terms of increased sense of pride, self-control and self-esteem.

When you have more willpower to do the things you want to do, it helps to reveal the much-needed self-control. The famous Marshmallow Test proved that self-control helps with success, better quality of life and happiness. Similarly, when you break your fast, your mind displays an unbelievable sense of gratefulness for food. It enhances the quality of life and nourishes your body.

Though more clinical studies are needed, it cannot be denied that intermittent fasting does help in a better quality of life. However, it is important to ensure you eat a healthy and wholesome diet during your eating window on the intermittent fasting plan. Since you get less time to eat, you will need to give more nutritional gains to your body when you eat.

CHAPTER FIVE:

Types of Intermittent Fasting

Intermittent fasting is the best way to improve your overall health and reach your fitness goals. For everything from giving you the required nutrition and reducing the risk of chronic diseases to weight loss and burning fat – intermittent fasting has proved its mettle in many ways. There are several types of intermittent fasts which can be implemented. We will be looking at the few popularly used and effective ones, such as:

- 16:8 method
- 5:2 method
- Eat-Stop-Eat
- Alternate-day fasting
- Warrior diet

16:8 Method

The 16:8 method (16 hours OFF and 8 hours ON) is also known as the daily window fasting. It is the easiest and the most popular intermittent fasting method followed by the majority. All you need to do is skip a meal! In this fasting method, you eat for 8 hours and fast for 16 hours. There are two ways of doing it:

- Skip breakfast and eat later in the day
- Or have an early dinner and don't eat anything until the next day (breakfast).

Some people do slight a bit of modification in the eating window, such as eating within one or 3 hours during the day and fast for 20 or 23 hours a day, i.e., 23:1 or 20:4 method. But when you fast for more than 20 hours, it is called the Warrior diet.

When you follow 16:8 fasting method, you eat within the 8-hour window (maybe, 11 a.m. – 7 p.m.) and then fast for the remaining 16 hours (7 p.m. until 11 a.m.). The fasting and eating window can vary depending on the individual. You can eat within a four-hour window or go for a seven-hour window, i.e., 20:4 or 17:7.

But the best choice would be to fast for 16 hours, which is inclusive of your sleeping hours. You can skip breakfast and have lunch as your first meal of the day and then finish the day with an early dinner. For instance, fast from 8 p.m. to 12 noon (16 hours – including sleep time) and have your first meal (lunch) at 12:30 p.m. and then dinner around 7 p.m. If you want, you can have snacks (fruit or veggies) around 4 p.m.

You can follow this method whenever you like – maybe twice a week or during the weekdays. You can also do it regularly for better results. When you are regular with this diet pattern, you get into the habit and your appetite also considerably reduces.

5:2 Method

This diet is the most popular intermittent fasting diet pattern as of now. It is also known as The Fast Diet. Michael Mosley, a British doctor and journalist, popularized this diet pattern.

It got its name - 5:2 diet - as you go on with your normal eating routine for five days and then restrict the calorie-intake for the remaining two days. You should only have 500-600 calories per day on those two days. You cannot call this a diet, as it is more of an eating pattern.

You don't find any restriction on what food you should eat, but it is more to do with when you should eat your food.

This is pretty easy – for five days a week, you just continue with your normal eating routine. No worries about restricting calories! You need to focus on the remaining two days of the week - the days when you should restrict your calorie consumption to 500 to 600 per day. (The math is 500 for women and 600 for men per day).

You can choose the two days as per your convenience, but the only thing to remember is you need to ensure you have a day's gap (non-fasting day) between the two days.

You can fast on Mondays and Wednesdays – 2 or 3 small meals on those two days with a check on the calories. The remaining days you can carry on with your regular food routine. However, it is important to eat the right food during the non-fasting days too – healthy, well-balanced, wholesome meals.

Eating processed food, meat, oily food, junk, etc. will not serve any purpose – as you will not be able to lose weight but on the contrary might put on more weight.

There shouldn't be too much of hogging or overeating on your non-fasting day – it should be the same quantity of food you eat normally. This dieting pattern is said to be the best to lose weight and improve your body's metabolic rate.

Eat-Stop-Eat

Eat-Stop-Eat aims to give the body a complete break from food for 24 hours. It is quite simple – you can fast once or maybe twice a week (depending on your routine). For instance, you can eat normally until 7 p.m. today and then fast until 7 p.m. the next day. You can then resume your normal eating routine (try sticking to the healthy and wholesome diet). You can repeat the fast after several days (after, maybe, two or three weeks).

One important thing to remember is - do not exceed two fasts in one week! Fasting once in a week should be more than enough, but if you feel you can manage with two, you can still go ahead!

You need to ensure your body is hydrated during your fasting days. You can have water, black coffee and herbal tea. In case you feel hungry, you can have a smoothie or cold-pressed fresh juice (without sugar or sweetener).

Similarly, when you break your fast, you can eat normally but ensure you don't indulge in overeating, as that would ruin the benefits of the fast. It is good to include a lot of vegetables, spices and fruit in your diet during your non-fasting days.

If you are following the Eat-Stop-Eat diet pattern to your regular routine, you can combine a consistent workout routine for your non-fasting days. But ensure you don't exercise on your fasting days as you might end up over-exerting your body muscles. This diet might cause headaches in some people.

Pregnant women, nursing mothers, people with diabetes or people with eating disorders should not observe this diet. You will need a good amount of self-control and should be able to decide which food will be good for you.

Alternate-day Fasting

Alternate day fasting or ADF is another type of intermittent fasting which works well for longevity and weight loss. The rules are quite simple – you fast alternate days, no calorie-intake should be present during your fast days, and you can eat normally during your eating days.

You can have only water during your fast days or can consume water and other fluids (black coffee, herbal tea, fresh juices, etc.), but none of the fluids should have sugar or sweetener added to them.

This fasting method has numerous benefits but only when it is done the right way. A healthy choice of food is more important. Combining exercise with your diet plan will be more effective towards your weight-loss goal as well as for your overall health. Ensure you don't eat processed food, as it might do no good to your health. Your food plate must have a combination of vegetables, fruit, spices and wholesome meal.

Most people will find this intermittent fasting method an easier choice, but some may find it difficult. People who eat more than three meals in a day might find it difficult. There are some who get irritated when they miss a meal – this pattern will not work for them either.

But again, it is fine! Each of us has our own individuality – the body metabolism, dietary choices, preferences and activity levels will be different.

The Warrior Diet

The Warrior diet is a combination of exercise and fasting. You will need to follow your gut feeling when it comes to choosing the right diet. Avoid getting tempted by processed food or junk food. Don't get too rigid with the types of macronutrients and calories that need to be consumed during the eating window. Instead, as the name implies, eat like a warrior! Our prehistoric warriors had little food during the day and had their meal at night, i.e., little food in the day and more food at night.

The Warrior diet is more to do with vigorous exercising (even during the fasting days) and controlled food-intake. You will need to exercise when your stomach is completely empty (preferably as soon as you wake up). You will have only one meal in a day. If you can adapt to this type of intermittent fasting, you will be able to burn more fat (into energy) and will get a lean physique without the need to count your calories.

Your exercise routine should be total body strength training – squats, pushups, pull-ups, high jumps, skipping and presses. You can also include high-intensity cardio exercises, such as frog jumps or sprints, in between these sessions. These sessions can last for between 20 and 45 minutes.

Since you can have only one meal in a day, you might take time to get adapted to this routine. You might feel weak or dizzy initially. Don't push it too hard! First, introduce your body to the diet routine gradually – maybe skip breakfast twice a week and eat your lunch and dinner as usual. Continue this for few weeks, then slowly skip two meals and get your body accustomed to the routine. Once your body is ready, get into the full-on warrior diet mode. Don't under-eat, eat normally during your non-fasting days. Include more whole, raw foods to enable your digestive enzymes to help you.

Since it is only one meal with a strong exercise regimen, you need to keep your body hydrated. Ensure you drink a lot of water and consume fluids like herbal tea, black coffee, fresh juice (cold-pressed) with no sugar or sweetener. You can also have green smoothies (without butter or cream). When you focus on drinking cold-pressed juices (from the whole food) or whole raw food, you are helping your body to reload, as these foods are full of enzymes.

Make sure you have a healthy organic, wholesome meal during your eating window. Add more vegetables, spices, greens and fruit to your plate. Drink enough water after your meal.

This diet might not be suitable for the general public as it might not fit into their daily lifestyles, work routines, body capacities, etc. Moreover, it is quite difficult to get all the required nutrients your body needs in just one meal every day.

Sometimes, this diet can leave you so hungry that you indulge in pigging the food, which will result in overeating. And this is definitely not going to help you lose weight. Similarly, not many people will be okay with exercising (especially strength training) on an empty stomach. They might feel dizzy and have a nauseous feeling.

It is, therefore, better to check with your physician before choosing this fasting method – or any method for that matter.

Listen to your body and choose the style that will best suit your routine. It should bring the best in your body's health making you feel energetic and lighter.

CHAPTER SIX:

Rules of Intermittent Fasting: What You Can and Cannot Eat or Drink

Now that you have a clear picture on what intermittent fasting is and the various benefits it imparts, you can get started with your dieting pattern. But before you begin intermittent fasting, it is advisable to understand what should and shouldn't be done. Avoid the common mistakes which people usually make when it comes to observing a fast.

The following is a list of do's and don'ts that you might have to adhere to while implementing intermittent fasting into your routine:

Do's:

Let your transition mode be slow

Ensure you don't get into intermittent fasting without understanding it clearly. Planning your diet pattern is important. You will need to research the different styles of intermittent fasting and choose the one that will best suit you. For instance, if you have planned to start with 16:8 diet, don't get into the 16 hours fasting window straightaway. Your body might be shocked because of the sudden change in routine. Start with a 12 hour fasting window and gradually increase it to 16 hours (during the next fast). Never get into the Eat-Stop-Eat protocol if fasting is completely new to you. Going without food for 24 hours might be difficult for you.

Listen to what your body has to say

When you start with intermittent fasting, try to listen to what your body has to say. Sometimes a particular fasting protocol might not suit your body. You might feel uncomfortable – continuous dizziness, nausea, frequent headaches, etc. Give your body some time to cope but if the symptoms are continuous, stop! Don't force your body. Accept that the particular intermittent fasting type doesn't suit your body.

Stay hydrated

Always ensure your body is hydrated during your fasting period. It doesn't mean that you cannot drink water when you are fasting. You need to avoid diet sodas or carbonated drinks because they might cause you dehydration. And technically speaking, they aren't recommended either.

Don'ts:

Avoid making yourself uncomfortable

If you are someone who is used to eating 4-6 small meals all through the day, then intermittent fasting can be tough on your body. You might feel tired and weak. Therefore, it is advisable to reduce the number of meals slowly before you implement intermittent fasting. In case you feel pale and weak during your fasting window, then it is time to change your intermittent fasting style. Choose a protocol that will suit your body as well as your lifestyle.

No overeating

A very common mistake most people make when they first observe intermittent fasting is – overeating. This happens because the eating window is short when compared to your fasting window. So, all you want to do is get your hands on anything and everything to eat. You might also end up eating too much junk food. This is not the right way to fast. Unhealthy eating will ruin all your effort. Stick to the routine normal diet you would usually have when you aren't fasting. Try to add more fruit, vegetables, spices, nuts, cereals, etc. to your food plate.

Don't keep watching the clock more than often

It is understandable that you would like to stick to your timing and ensure that your eating window starts at the right time. But don't overreact. Prepare your mind to accept that food needs to be eaten during a specific time period. Be clear on how often your food intake should happen. Set a timer on your mobile to help you.

Rules on what to eat or drink

The general rule of thumb is – drinking anything with less than 50 calories is allowed during your fasting period. This is because drinking or eating anything within 50 calories will still let your body remain in the fasted state.

You can eat or drink the following during your **fasting window**:

- Plain water
- Fruit (Half or one)
- Fresh cold-pressed juice (without sugar or sweeteners)
- Green smoothies (without dairy or cream)

You can eat or drink the following during your **eating window**:

- Raw or cooked vegetables
- Fruit
- Cereals
- Spices
- Nuts

- Wholesome meal (whole food with vegetables and spices)
- Brown rice, Whole multigrain bread, etc
- Smoothies (Fruit or Vegetable)
- Cold-pressed juices
- Plain water

You cannot eat or drink the following during your **fasting window**:

- Flavored drinks
- Diet Coke
- Carbonated drinks
- Pastries
- Sugar-rich drink or food, etc

You cannot eat or drink the following during your **eating window**:

- Processed food
- Junk snacks
- Oily food
- Alcohol
- Sugar-rich food
- Too much dairy
- Red meat, etc

Generic rules of Intermittent Fasting

Most of the rules that are mentioned below are clear and straightforward. It is up to you to stick to these rules and get out of your usual routine. This will help you acquire the required benefits from intermittent fasting.

- If you want to make intermittent fasting your new habit, then you will need to take things slowly. It is important to give your body the required time to adapt to the new nutritional style. It takes 66 days to develop a habit. So, start fasting for 1-2 days a week and then gradually increase it to 3-4 days in a week.

- Exercising when you are in a fasted state will help your body lose more fat. This is because your blood sugar levels are at their lowest. Listen to your body. If you feel your body cannot handle strength-training, stick to simple exercises for 30-45 minutes – maybe, muscle stretches, yoga, walking, etc.

- Don't stress yourself by preparing the meal at the start of the eating window. Instead, get your meal ready much earlier so that you can straightaway start having your food at the start of your eating window.

- Keep yourself completely occupied when you are fasting. If you have more free time during your fasting window, you end up feeling hungrier, or you keep thinking about food. Instead, if you are busy, you will feel that time is running faster.

- Your body should be completely hydrated during the fasting period. Keep drinking loads of water. You can also have herbal tea or black coffee occasionally. Have fresh juices without sugar. Adding sugar will deter all the benefits of fasting.

- Don't keep standing on that weighing machine every single day. Fasting is going to reboot your body's system and bring back insulin sensitivity. And this process doesn't happen overnight. So, give it time. Remember, each day you successfully complete the fast is a victory. It takes you a step closer to your goal.

- Listen to your body. Know your limits. Don't overexert. It might take some time to get adapted to intermittent fasting. Start fasting for 12 hours first, then stretch another hour next time, and then another. Finally get to your target of 16 hours fasting window.

- Every time you successfully finish a fast, congratulate yourself. Feast on your favorite dish after the fast (but ensure it is a healthy diet).

When you start intermittent fasting, it feels like you are clicking a turbo switch. The moment the switch is on, everything starts to accelerate. You lose fat, your metabolic rate increases and finally you get a lean physique. All said and done, if you don't stick to your plans, then you end up ruining all your effort. Ensure you get the right meal plan done and adhere to it.

CHAPTER SEVEN:

Getting Started

As mentioned in the previous chapter, don't rush into things. Take it slow. Allow your body to understand the new diet regimen. After you decide the type of intermittent fasting you are going to start with, show a trial session to your body. Let's say you are going to start with 16:8 fasting approach. Prepare your body by following the steps mentioned below:

First Day –Don't eat anything after dinner

- Go ahead with your usual eating routine
- But once you have eaten your dinner, stop eating.
- When you have your dinner around 7 p.m., it is natural to feel hungry by 9 or 10 p.m. You then get comfortable on your couch in front of the TV with a bag of potato chips or popcorn. Don't do this!
- Drink a glass of water or maybe, have a cup of herbal tea.
- Get to bed early. Sleeping is the best way to put an end to this.

Second Day – Have late breakfast

- Congratulations! You just completed a 12-hour fast
- You had your dinner at 7 p.m., and now it is 7 a.m. You successfully resisted your temptation to have food after dinner.
- 12 hours eating and 12 hours fasting is a good start for your body

- Wasn't it easy? When you sleep, time flies! Let the maximum time of your fasting window, be your sleep time.
- Have black coffee or herbal tea after you brush your teeth.
- Delay your breakfast, maybe, to 10 a.m. (best time!)
- Since you delayed your breakfast, your lunchtime needs to be delayed, as you won't feel hungry. So, lunchtime may be, 2 p.m.
- Finish your day by having dinner at 7 p.m.

Follow the steps you did on your first day and again continue the routine by delaying your breakfast (until 10 a.m., maybe!)

Third day – Stop snacking!

Well done, you just completed a 15-hour fasting window (7 p.m. to 10 a.m.). Yesterday, you might have had some snacks after lunch.

Today, avoid eating anything between your lunch and dinner. No snacks! Drink lots of water or maybe have fresh juice (cold-pressed) without sugar. Keep yourself busy so that you don't feel like wanting to munch some snacks.

Follow the routine – dinner at 7 p.m., no food after dinner, have late breakfast at 10 a.m. next day and no snacking between meals.

Fourth day – Time to skip breakfast.

Bravo! You successfully completed a 15-hour fasting window and had only three meals during your eating window (no snacks!)

Today, it is time for you to skip your breakfast. Let your first meal of the day be at 11 a.m. Have your lunch at 11 a.m., don't snack until dinner time (7 p.m.) Drink lots of water in between meals.

Continue with your routine again: dinner at 7 p.m., no food after dinner, skip breakfast, no snacking between lunch and dinner.

Fifth day – Get to the repeat mode.

Wow! You just successfully completed your 16-hour fasting window. Dinner at 7 p.m. last night, no breakfast, first meal at 11 a.m.., no snacks in between until 7 P.M.

You have now successfully started with your 16:8 intermittent fasting routine. Your eating window is now reduced to 8 hours, and fasting window has increased to 16 hours.

Now that you have understood how to start with the intermittent fasting routine, you can now chart down the days you would like to implement them. To begin with, you can do it for 2 days in a week and then slowly increase it to 4 or 5 days.

CHAPTER EIGHT:

Frequently Asked Questions

Is it good if I exercise during my fasting window?

Yes! It is good if you can combine a variety of exercises in your workout routine when you fast. Exercising during the fasting period helps to burn more fat than usual. Yoga and walking can compliment your intermittent fasting better.

You might notice your energy levels going a little low and this is because your body uses your glycogen reserves. Instead of exercising for a longer period, it is advisable to exercise for shorter durations. Maybe you can try a high-intensity workout regimen for 20 to 30 minutes during your fasting days.

Is it normal to feel hungry when you observe intermittent fasting?

Since you are not eating any food for a continuous period of time (which is not your usual routine), your stomach might keep growling here and there. Ghrelin, the hunger hormone, will get triggered and tell your brain that you are starving. But your body adjusts to the routine after two or three fasts.

Why do I get a headache during the days I fast?

Not everyone gets a headache. Research was done on headache symptoms with people who observe fasting on Ramadan. Mostly women are prone to headaches during the fasting period. The findings don't link it to dehydration, but researchers feel that it might be withdrawal symptoms.

It usually goes away after the first few fasts but to relieve yourself from the pain, you can treat it the normal way. Get some fresh air and drink lots of water during your fasting period.

How frequently should I observe intermittent fasting?

There is no hard-and-fast rule. It basically depends on your body and the routine. You can observe the 24-hour fast once in a week. But in a case where your body can manage it, you can do it twice a week. But don't go beyond two fasts in a week.

Can I have one or two fruit in between meals during the eating window?

Yes! You can eat whatever you want during your eating window. It is not necessary that you should stick to two meals or three meals in your eating window. You can eat whenever you want during that period. For instance, have your lunch at 1 p.m., then snack on a fruit at 4 p.m. and have an early dinner at 7 p.m.

It depends on your routine – some people prefer to have two good meals during their eating windows while some will want to stick to their three or four meal routine in that 8-hour eating period.

Remember, you are not fasting between your meals. You are fasting after your meals.

CONCLUSION

And with that, we have come to the end of the book. Thank you once again for choosing the book.

The book has covered the primary objective, which is to act as a beginner's guide to readers who would like to know more about intermittent fasting. The book also gives a quick overview of the role of intermittent fasting in weight loss, burning fat, maintaining a healthy body and improving lifespan.

It is crucial to listen to your body and choose the fasting protocol that best suits your lifestyle, work routine and eating habits. For effective results, combine your intermittent fasting method with a good workout regimen.

I sincerely hope this book was useful and has helped in answering most of the questions you had in mind. Thanks for reading!

SOURCES

https://idmprogram.com/fasting-a-history-part-i/

http://www.rawfoodexplained.com/introduction-to-fasting/what-is-fasting.html

https://www.perfectketo.com/guide/intermittent-fasting/

https://www.lifehack.org/articles/lifestyle/intermittent-fasting-the-ultimate-weight-loss-hack.html

https://www.dietvsdisease.org/intermittent-fasting-is-powerful-for-weight-loss/

http://www.nowloss.com/intermittent-fasting-diet-plan.htm

https://medium.com/@drbradysalcido/6-surprising-brain-power-benefits-of-intermittent-fasting-49ad1bc39e04

https://drjockers.com/fasting-improves-brain-function/

http://www.afr.com/business/health/intermittent-fasting-affects-your-body-and-brain-in-surprising-ways-20180322-h0xusu

https://shinedrink.com/blogs/brainbites/the-effects-of-intermittent-fasting-on-brain-function

https://www.thomasdelauer.com/how-to-use-fasting-for-inflammation-and-longevity-benefits-of-intermittent-fasting/

https://www.healthline.com/health/fasting-and-cancer#research

https://hope4cancer.com/blog/healing-cancer-on-time-how-intermittent-fasting-may-help/

https://www.homecuresthatwork.com/21144/intermittent-fasting-reverses-diabetes/

http://www.beliefnet.com/wellness/health/6-health-benefits-of-intermittent-fasting.aspx?p=8

https://www.perfectketo.com/16-8-intermittent-fasting-ketosis/

https://www.dietdoctor.com/lose-weight-using-intermittent-fasting

https://www.healthline.com/nutrition/the-5-2-diet-guide#section7

https://www.livestrong.com/article/438695-how-eat-stop-eat-works/

https://www.livestrong.com/article/83394-start-warrior-diet/

https://www.perfectketo.com/guide/intermittent-fasting/

https://www.globalhealingcenter.com/natural-health/alternate-day-fasting/

https://www.myoleanfitness.com/intermittent-fasting-what-to-eat-drink/

https://healthylivinglab.com/dos-donts-intermittent-fasting/

https://mindfulketo.com/how-to-start-fasting/

https://yurielkaim.com/how-to-do-intermittent-fasting/

https://jamesclear.com/reader-mailbag-intermittent-fasting

http://www.barbrothersgroningen.com/intermittent-fasting-plan/